SCIATIC WORKOUT

FOR BEGINNERS

A Comprehensive Guide To Relieve, Restore, Strengthen And Alleviating Sciatic Pain Through Targeted Exercises

LAMBERT FETTERMAN

DISCLAIMER

The content in this book is offered only for general informative purposes. While every effort has been taken to guarantee the content's accuracy and completeness, the author and publisher accept no responsibility for any mistakes or omissions, or for the results of using the information given herein. The methods, recommendations, and directions in this book are not guaranteed to be appropriate for every person, and readers should exercise caution and seek professional counsel if required before undertaking any of the projects or techniques detailed in this book.

Table of Contents

CHAPTER 1

Understanding Sciatic Pain

What Is Sciatica?

Sciatica is discomfort that radiates down the sciatic nerve, which runs from your lower back to your hips, buttocks, and down each leg. It is often caused by sciatic nerve compression or inflammation, resulting in pain, numbness, or tingling sensations along its route. Understanding the condition's underlying origins and symptoms is critical for successful treatment.

Causes Of Sciatic Pain

Herniated discs, bone spurs, spinal stenosis, and even muscle disorders like piriformis syndrome may all cause sciatic discomfort.

These underlying conditions often cause sciatic nerve compression or irritation, resulting in pain that varies in degree and duration.

Symptoms And Identification

Recognizing sciatic pain's characteristic symptoms, which may include shooting pain that spreads from the lower back to the legs, numbness or tingling sensations in the afflicted leg, weakness in the leg or foot, and even difficulties moving the affected limb, is essential for identifying it. When sitting, sneezing, or coughing, these symptoms may aggravate.

Understanding the nature of sciatic pain is critical for building methods for managing and alleviating discomfort, especially for novices searching for alleviation activities.

CHAPTER 2

Foundations Of Exercise And Sciatica

Sciatica, which is often caused by sciatic nerve compression or irritation, may cause pain, tingling, or numbness along the route of this nerve, commonly spreading from the lower back down into the leg. Exercises are essential for controlling sciatic pain, assisting with healing, and increasing mobility. Understanding the fundamentals of sciatica exercises is critical for properly treating this ailment.

Importance Of Exercise In Managing Sciatic Pain

Regular exercise is essential for relieving and controlling sciatica. Specific exercises may help reduce sciatic nerve irritation, strengthen supporting muscles, and increase flexibility. They also improve posture and general spinal health, lowering the probability of repeated attacks of sciatica.

Guidelines For Safe Workouts With Sciatica

When dealing with sciatica, it's important to exercise carefully and under supervision, particularly during the acute period. Avoid activities that cause discomfort and instead concentrate on soft motions that do not strain the back or irritate the damaged nerve. Gradual progression and consistency are essential for adapting the body to exercise without generating extra pain.

Benefits Of Specific Exercises

Several exercises are available to help with sciatic pain treatment and management. Stretching, strengthening, and low-impact activities help improve flexibility, spine stability, and sciatic nerve strain. These exercises concentrate on the lower back, hips, and legs, providing both short-term pain alleviation and long-term advantages by treating the underlying causes of sciatica.

Would you want to go further into certain exercises or investigate any specific forms of sciatica workouts?

CHAPTER 3

Preparation And Warm-Up

Importance Of Warm-Up
For Sciatic Workouts

It is essential to thoroughly prepare your body before participating in any sort of activity targeted at relieving sciatic pain. Warm-ups are essential for preparing your muscles, improving blood flow, and lowering your chance of injury during exercises. Warm-up activities are especially important for those suffering from sciatica owing to the sensitivity and susceptibility of the afflicted region.

Pre-Exercise Stretches For Sciatic Relief

Begin with mild stretches that target the afflicted regions of sciatic discomfort. These stretches are designed to release stiff muscles, especially those in the lower back, buttocks, and legs, which are along the route of the sciatic nerve.

1. Begin on all fours, arch your back like a cat, then dip your spine down, lifting your head and tailbone (cow posture). For spine flexibility, repeat this exercise while synchronizing it with your breath.

2. Knee-to-Chest Stretch: While lying on your back, raise one knee to your chest and hold it there with both hands for 15-30

seconds. Stretch both sides by alternating legs.

3. Cross one leg over the other knee while sitting or lying down, then slowly draw the crossed leg toward your chest.

4. Stretch your hamstrings by extending one leg forward and leaning forward, attempting to touch your toes while maintaining your back straight.

5. Kneel on the floor, then sit back on your heels, dropping your upper body to rest on or between your thighs and extending your arms forward.

Mindfulness Techniques For Pain Management

Individuals suffering from sciatica may benefit from mindfulness techniques in addition to physical stretches and warm-ups. Techniques such as regulated breathing, meditation, or guided imagery may help to calm the mind and body before participating in workouts, reducing the severity of sciatic pain.

Deep, regulated breathing techniques may assist in soothing the nervous system and alleviate tension in the afflicted muscles. Mindfulness meditation practices promote concentrating on the present moment, distancing oneself from discomfort, and cultivating a feeling of serenity.

These first procedures are critical in establishing an ideal atmosphere for future sciatic exercises. They not only improve the efficiency of the workouts, but they also lower the risk of exacerbating the ailment and promote general well-being. Before beginning any new fitness plan, always see a healthcare expert, particularly if you have a condition like sciatica.

CHAPTER 4

Low-Impact Exercises For Sciatic Relief

Sciatica, which is characterized by pain radiating down the route of the sciatic nerve, may be relieved with specific low-impact activities. Incorporating these exercises into your program will help relieve sciatic discomfort while also improving general flexibility and strength.

Stretching And Strengthening The Lower Back

• **Child's Pose Stretch:** Sit on your heels, raise your arms forward, and drop your chest toward the ground in this yoga-inspired stretch. This helps to lengthen and extend the lower back, relieving the sciatic nerve.

• Cat-Cow Stretch: Begin on your hands and knees, arching your back upward (the "cat") then lowering your back while elevating your head (the "cow" posture). This dynamic stretch improves spine flexibility and may reduce sciatic pain.

Gentle Yoga Poses For Sciatica

• Downward-Facing Dog: Begin on your hands and knees, then elevate your hips toward the ceiling in an inverted V shape. This position stretches the hamstrings and lower back, perhaps relieving sciatic nerve strain.

• **Pigeon Pose:** From a sitting posture, stretch one leg behind you and pull one knee forward, sinking into a forward bend over the bent leg. The pigeon position focuses on the hips and helps relieve sciatica stress.

Core Strengthening Exercises

• **Pelvic Tilts:** Lie down on your back with your legs bent and your feet flat on the floor. Engage your core muscles as you gently tilt your pelvis upward. This exercise helps to stabilize the lower back and promotes the health of the sciatic nerve.

• **Bridge Exercise:** Lie on your back and raise your hips toward the ceiling, making a straight line from your shoulders to your knees. This strengthens the core and glutes, providing lower back stability.

Incorporating these low-impact exercises into your regimen while paying attention to your body's cues may help beginners achieve sciatic relief. Before beginning a new fitness plan, always speak with a healthcare practitioner, particularly if you have pre-existing health concerns.

CHAPTER 5

Cardio And Sciatic Health

Cardiovascular workouts are important for general health, including the management of sciatic pain. Low-impact aerobic exercises help to improve blood circulation, reduce inflammation, and promote general well-being. Certain cardiac workouts are especially good for those suffering from sciatica since they do not aggravate the problem.

Low-Impact Cardiovascular Exercises

1. Swimming: Water-based workouts, such as swimming or aqua aerobics, provide a weightless environment that relieves strain

on the spine while developing muscles. These exercises stimulate the whole body without putting the sciatic nerve under strain.

2. Elliptical training provides for a flowing movement that is mild on the lower back and sciatic nerve. It gives you a full-body exercise without the jarring effect of other types of cardio.

3. Cycling: Stationary or recumbent cycling might be beneficial for those suffering from sciatica. It is a low-impact workout that improves leg muscles and increases flexibility without putting pressure on the lower back.

Stationary Cycling And Sciatic Relief

Individuals suffering from sciatica might benefit from regulated and regular exercise on stationary bikes. Proper bike placement is critical, ensuring that the seat height and handlebar position are comfortable and compatible with the body's natural posture. Begin with a low degree of resistance and progressively raise it as your comfort and strength improve.

Cycling's repetitive action helps to stretch and strengthen the muscles around the lower back and legs. It also helps with flexibility, which may help relieve sciatic nerve strain.

Walking Techniques For Sciatica

Walking is a simple but effective sciatic treatment workout. To avoid exacerbating the problem, proper walking methods are required:

• **Stance:** While walking, maintain an upright stance. Ascertain that your head is up, your shoulders are back, and your spine is in a neutral posture.

• **Stride Length:** Do not overstride. Shorter, more comfortable steps, landing on your heels and moving through your feet to softly push off.

• Terrain: Choose flat, even surfaces to reduce impact. Avoid uneven or difficult terrain that may strain your back.

• Shoes: Put on supportive and comfy shoes with enough arch support and cushioning for your feet.

Regular, regular low-impact cardiovascular workouts may help manage sciatica while also improving overall physical health.

CHAPTER 6

Balance And Stability Exercises

Importance Of Balance For Sciatica

Maintaining balance is essential for dealing with sciatica pain. It strengthens the muscles that support the spine and hips, relieving strain on the sciatic nerve and improving posture.

Exercises To Improve Stability And Prevent Injury

1. Single-Leg Stands: Stand on one leg while bending the other leg slightly at the knee. If necessary, grab a chair or a wall for

support. This assists in engaging core muscles and improving stability.

2. Lie on your back with your knees bent and your feet flat on the floor for bridges. Engage your glutes and core muscles to lift your hips off the ground. Hold for a few seconds before lowering back down. This exercise strengthens and stabilizes the spine by strengthening the lower back and gluteal muscles.

3. Planks: Form a straight line from head to heels by supporting your body on your elbows and toes. Engage your core and maintain the posture while keeping your back flat. Planks improve total core stability, which helps with sciatic pain treatment.

4. **Balancing on Unstable Surfaces:** Challenge your balance by standing on a foam pad or cushion. This enhances proprioception and strengthens the stabilizing muscles.

Proprioception Training For Sciatic Health

1. **Balance Boards or Wobble Boards:** Using a balance board or wobble board tests balance and proprioception, which benefits the muscles that support the spine and hips.

2. **Tai Chi or Qigong:** These activities stress slow, methodical motions that develop balance, flexibility, and coordination, all of which may help with sciatica.

3. Yoga and Pilates: Specific yoga positions and Pilates exercises emphasize balance, core strength, and flexibility, all of which lead to improved stability and decreased sciatic discomfort.

Incorporating these exercises into a fitness regimen regularly helps to improve balance, stability, and general posture, which contributes considerably to controlling and avoiding sciatic pain. Before beginning any fitness program, always see a healthcare practitioner, particularly if you have sciatica or other health problems.

CHAPTER 7

Mind-Body Practices For Pain Management

Meditation And Relaxation Techniques

Meditation entails concentrating one's attention and relaxing one's thoughts. It helps to reduce stress and tension, which may aggravate sciatic pain. Guided meditation, mindfulness practices, or deep breathing methods may help relieve pain by encouraging relaxation and relieving muscle tension.

Breathing Exercises For Sciatic Relief

Focused breathing exercises, such as diaphragmatic breathing or yoga Pranayama methods, may aid in relaxation and stress reduction. Controlled breathing also improves oxygenation and circulation, which may help alleviate sciatic pain.

Visualization And Positive Affirmations

Visualization methods include mentally imagining serene, pain-free environments. These activities, when combined with positive affirmations, which concentrate on happy thoughts and words, may help shift attention away from pain and foster a good mood, possibly lowering the feeling of sciatic pain.

Mind-Body Practices Have Many Advantages

• **Stress Management:** Stress may increase pain perception. Mind-body techniques help to control pain by lowering stress hormones.

• **Enhanced Relaxation:** These approaches produce a relaxation response, which calms the body and reduces tension, both of which may contribute to sciatic pain.

• **Better Mental State:** They lead to a more positive mental attitude, which may help with chronic pain issues such as sciatica.

Including Mind-Body Practices

• Consistency: Regular practice improves the efficacy of these strategies. It is good to begin with short sessions and progressively increase length.

• Integration: When mind-body practices are combined with other exercises and therapies, they may give complete pain alleviation and total well-being.

• Professional Guidance: To guarantee perfect technique and enhance efficacy, beginners may benefit from guided sessions or workshops taught by experienced teachers.

Individuals may not only manage discomfort but also encourage relaxation, decrease tension, and create a positive mentality conducive to general well-being by adding these mind-body activities into a sciatic exercise program.

CHAPTER 8

Incorporating Lifestyle Changes

Ergonomics And Posture Improvement

Poor posture and ergonomics may cause sciatic pain. Making changes to how you sit, stand, and move may greatly reduce your pain.

• **Proper Sitting Posture:** While sitting, keep your spine neutral. To relieve tension, use a cushion or lumbar roll to support the lower back.

• **Standing Techniques:** Avoid standing for lengthy periods. If you must stand for a lengthy amount of time, distribute your weight evenly between your legs, wear supportive footwear, and use an anti-fatigue mat.

• Lifting Techniques: When lifting, bend at the knees, maintain your spine straight, and lift using your legs rather than your back.

• Workstation Ergonomics: To improve excellent posture and prevent strain, adjust desk height, and chair position, and monitor height.

Dietary Considerations For Sciatic Health

Certain foods and minerals may either stimulate or relieve inflammation, which may have an impact on sciatic pain.

• **Anti-Inflammatory Diet:** To decrease inflammation, include foods high in omega-3 fatty acids, such as salmon, walnuts, and flaxseeds.

• **Hydration:** Drink enough water to keep your spine's discs hydrated and flexible.

• **Avoid Trigger Foods:** For some people, eliminating processed foods, excessive coffee, and foods heavy in refined sugars provides relief.

Sleep And Its Impact On Sciatic Pain

Quality sleep is essential for general health, including the management of sciatica.

• **Sleeping Positions:** Experiment with various sleeping positions to find one that relieves lower back pressure and lowers sciatic discomfort.

• **Mattress and Pillow Support:** Use a medium-firm mattress that maintains your spine's natural curve. Use a suitable cushion to support your head and neck.

• Establish a peaceful nighttime ritual to increase sleep quality. Consider meditation or mild stretches before going to bed.

Changes In General Lifestyle

• **Regular Exercise:** To maintain flexibility and develop supporting muscles, engage in low-impact activities such as swimming, walking, or yoga.

• **Stress Reduction and Mindfulness:** Stress may aggravate discomfort. Mindfulness, meditation, and deep breathing techniques might assist in regulating stress, perhaps lowering sciatic pain.

• **Avoid Prolonged Sitting or Standing:** Alternate between sitting, standing, and walking throughout the day to avoid sciatic nerve stiffness and pressure.

Individuals suffering from sciatic pain may dramatically improve their comfort and general well-being by making these lifestyle adjustments. Before making significant changes to your lifestyle or workout regimen, always see a healthcare practitioner, particularly if you have a medical condition like sciatica.

CHAPTER 9

Recovery And Rehabilitation

Cooling Down After Workouts

It is essential to cool down after exercising to lessen muscular tension and avoid damage. Gentle stretching or relaxation exercises may help progressively lower heart rate and return muscles to a resting condition.

• **Stretching Routines:** Post-exercise stretches that target the lower back and legs help relieve stress and avoid stiffness. Concentrate on mild stretches that lengthen muscles without straining them.

• **Breathing and Relaxation:** Techniques such as deep breathing exercises or progressive muscle relaxation may help to calm the nervous system and reduce muscular tension caused by sciatic pain.

Recovery Periods: Adequate rest between exercises is essential for the body to recover and rebuild. Allowing the body enough time to heal is critical for anyone dealing with sciatica. This might include a mix of rest days, mild activity, and maintaining enough sleep.

• **Alternate exercises:** On rest days, mild exercises like walking, swimming, or moderate yoga (if permitted) may improve blood circulation and aid recuperation without putting too much pressure on the sciatic nerve.

Professional Help And Rehabilitation

Seeking advice from healthcare specialists like physical therapists or chiropractors might be useful. They may give individualized rehabilitation plans, suitable exercises, and hands-on therapies to alleviate sciatic pain.

• **Physical Therapy:** A physical therapist may create a personalized exercise program that progressively increases strength, flexibility, and stability in the afflicted regions.

Targeted stretches, core strengthening, and posture correction may be included in these workouts.

- Chiropractic Care: Chiropractors may perform spinal adjustments and manipulations to relieve sciatic nerve irritation. They may also recommend additional modalities such as ultrasound or electrical stimulation to help with pain reduction and recovery.

Remember that everyone's experience with sciatica is unique, so it's critical to work with a healthcare practitioner to design a safe and effective exercise plan tailored to your requirements and limits.

CHAPTER 10

Long-Term Maintenance And Prevention

Strategies For Preventing Sciatic Pain

Sciatic discomfort is often caused by underlying disorders such as spinal misalignment, herniated discs, or muscular stress. Among the preventative measures are:

• **Maintain Good Posture:** Poor posture may aggravate sciatica. Use ergonomics at work, supportive seats, and maintain proper posture when sitting and standing.

• Maintain a regular workout routine that focuses on core strength, flexibility, and back muscles. Avoid abrupt, vigorous actions that cause back pain.

• **Maintaining a Healthy Weight:** Excess weight puts strain on the spine, which contributes to sciatica. A healthy diet and regular exercise aid in weight management, minimizing tension on the spine.

• **Mindful Lifting Techniques:** Lift heavy things with your knees bent and your back straight to avoid straining your spine and sciatic nerve.

• **normal Footwear:** To preserve normal alignment and decrease strain on the lower back and legs, wear supportive shoes with enough arch support.

Maintaining A Healthy Exercise Routine

Regular physical exercise is essential for keeping your back healthy and avoiding sciatica. The following are some essential exercises and practices:

• **Stretching regimen:** Establish a regular stretching regimen that focuses on the hamstrings, piriformis, and lower back. Stretching regularly increases flexibility and removes strain on the sciatic nerve.

• **Strength Training:** Include activities that improve your core, back and legs. Pilates, yoga, and particular strength training activities help improve spine stability and support.

• **Low-Impact Exercises:** Participate in low-impact activities like swimming, walking, or cycling. These exercises improve blood flow, muscular flexibility, and spinal health overall.

• **Mind-Body Practices:** Yoga, tai chi, and meditation may help regulate stress, which frequently leads to muscular tightness and aggravates sciatic pain.

Lifestyle Adjustments For Long-Term Relief

Certain lifestyle adjustments may considerably help with long-term sciatic pain relief:

• **Ergonomic Work Environment:** Ensure that your workstation is ergonomically constructed. Adjust the height of your chair, utilize sufficient lumbar support, and take frequent pauses to stretch and move about.

• **Proper Sleep Posture:** Select a sleeping posture that promotes the spine's natural curve. Use pillows for extra support, particularly if you sleep on your side.

• **Regular Visits to Healthcare Providers:** Visiting a physical therapist, chiropractor, or orthopedic expert regularly may assist in monitoring your back health and giving preventative treatment.

• **Mindfulness and Stress Reduction:** Mindfulness, meditation, and relaxation practices may help relieve stress, which can increase sciatic symptoms.

Incorporating these activities into your daily routine will help you maintain spinal health, reduce your risk of sciatic pain, and improve your overall well-being. Before beginning any new fitness plan, always speak with a healthcare provider, particularly if you have underlying health concerns.

Conclusion

Understanding and controlling sciatica with specific exercises is an important step toward relieving pain and recovering mobility. Combating sciatic pain via exercise is a lifelong struggle that demands patience, perseverance, and a conscious attitude.

Finally, this beginner's guide has provided you with the necessary core information and exercises to properly manage sciatic pain. However, it's important to note that each person's sciatica experience is unique, and obtaining expert assistance or guidance from healthcare specialists is critical.

You may progressively strengthen and support the lower back while limiting the strain on the sciatic nerve by including low-impact activities such as stretching, strengthening, and carefully planned aerobic routines into your daily routine.

Consistency and patience are essential; although progress may be slow, the aim is to increase flexibility, decrease discomfort, and improve general mobility. Pay attention to your body and alter activities as required to prevent worsening pain.

Finally, it is critical to maintain a comprehensive approach to health. Along with exercises, consider adopting healthy lifestyle habits such as correct diet, enough hydration, stress management strategies, and adequate rest to improve overall well-being and assist in the successful treatment of sciatic pain.

While these exercises might be useful, it is important to contact a healthcare expert before beginning any new fitness plan, particularly if you have a specific health problem such as sciatica.

Maintain your attention to your health, and you will see major gains in controlling and

minimizing sciatic pain with these exercises
with time and perseverance.

THE END